NAVIGATING TRANSIENT ISCHEMIC ATTACK WITH CONFIDENCE AND CARE

Empowering And Transformative Strategies For Controlling Blood Pressure And Mental Health

DR. WESLEY IAN

DISCLAIMER

The information in this book is not meant to replace professional medical advice, diagnosis, or treatment; rather, it is meant mainly for general informational reasons. If you have any questions about a medical problem, you should always consult your doctor or another trained health expert. Don't ever discount expert medical advice or put off getting it because of something you've read in this book.

Any negative effects or repercussions arising from the usage of the material provided herein are not the responsibility of the book's author or publisher. It should be noted by readers that the material in this book is not all-inclusive and might not address every facet of the subject. Furthermore, new research may have an impact on how health concerns are understood or treated because medical knowledge is always changing.

No particular test, treatment, method, or product mentioned in this book is endorsed or promoted by the author or publisher. The reader assumes all risk associated with using the information included in this book.

Before making any big decisions regarding your health, it's crucial to speak with a licensed healthcare provider. The relationship between a patient and their healthcare practitioner should not be replaced by this book, nor is it meant to offer medical advice.

The opinions presented in this book are the author's and may not necessarily represent those of the publisher. Any errors, omissions, or inaccuracies in the information in this book are not the responsibility of the author or publisher.

It is recommended that readers independently confirm any information contained in this book and speak with a healthcare provider about their specific medical needs and state of health.

TABLE OF CONTENTS

ABOUT THE BOOK

The book "Navigating Transient Ischemic Attack with Confidence and Care" serves as a thorough manual to help people understand the complicated world of transient epidemic attacks (TIAs). This book's significance rests in its capacity to arm readers with information, tactics, and a proactive mindset for handling and averting TIAs. The opening chapter establishes a relationship with the reader right away by extending a kind welcome and outlining the goal of the book.

An in-depth discussion of the TIA definition, causes, symptoms, and the vital significance of early detection is provided in introductory section. This background information provides context for the upcoming chapters and lays a strong basis for readers to understand the lifestyle and medical elements of TIAs.

The medical terrain surrounding transient ischemic attacks (TIAs) is explored. The reader is educated on diagnosis, distinguishing TIAs from strokes, seeking medical advice, and treatment options. This medical knowledge is essential for making well-informed decisions and working well with healthcare providers.

The book goes one step further in demonstrating the value of lifestyle changes in preventing TIAs. This includes recommendations for moderation in alcohol consumption and smoking, as well as guidance for food, exercise, and stress management. These lifestyle changes make a big difference in the overall approach to TIA management.

The topic is medication management, with an explanation of the several drugs that can be used to treat TIA. An extensive review of blood pressure control, cholesterol-lowering drugs, and ant platelet and anticoagulant drugs is given in this section. A thorough comprehension of these pharmacological therapies is essential for anyone looking to properly manage their disease.

Beyond the physical discusses the psychological and emotional difficulties related to TIAs. The comprehensive discussion of coping mechanisms, support networks, and mental health issues acknowledges the interconnectedness of health and wellness.

Building a thorough care plan and educating readers are the main goals of chapters six and seven. Proactive approaches to TIA management stress education on the condition, keeping up with research advancements, and actively advocating for one's health.

The book addresses the inevitable obstacles and failures, offering helpful guidance on handling difficulties, adjusting daily routines, and building mental toughness and resilience. With its painstakingly written chapters, this extensive book is a source of empowerment and knowledge for anybody traversing the treacherous path of transient epidemic attacks."

CHAPTER ONE

INTRODUCTION TO TRANSIENT ISCHEMIC ATTACK

RECOGNIZING TRANSIENT ISCHEMIC ATTACK

Transient Ischemic Attack (TIA): Often called a "mini-stroke," TIA is a medical condition that requires careful attention because it may indicate more serious cerebrovascular events. This introduction explores the definition, causes, symptoms, and critical importance of early detection of TIA.

SYNOPSIS AND DEFINITION

An acronym for transient ischemic attack (TIA) is "transient disruption of blood flow to the brain leading to transient neurological symptoms." Although brief, TIAs can be a warning sign of an upcoming stroke and emphasize the critical need for prompt medical attention. The term "ischemic" denotes that the cause is a temporary restriction of blood supply, frequently brought on by a blood clot or plaque in the arteries leading to the brain.

REASONS AND DANGER FACTORS

Gaining an understanding of the etiology and risk factors of transient ischemic attacks is crucial to appreciating the complexity of this condition. One of the main causes is the development of emboli, or blood clots, which block blood vessels in the brain and cause a temporary decrease in blood flow. Atherosclerosis, a condition marked by the accumulation of fatty deposits in the arteries, is a major risk factor for the formation of these clots. Other risk factors include age, smoking, hypertension, diabetes, and age, with those over 55 being at a higher risk.

SIGNS OF CONCERN AND SYMPTOMS

Understanding the signs and symptoms of a transient ischemic attack (TIA) is essential for timely medical attention. TIA symptoms are transient and can include sudden disorientation, trouble speaking or understanding speech, loss of balance or coordination, vision problems, and facial drooping. Although TIA symptoms typically go away quickly, they should not be disregarded as they could indicate a more serious stroke.

Being aware of these warning signs can help people and medical professionals act quickly, potentially preventing additional brain damage.

THE VALUE OF EARLY IDENTIFICATION

The significance of early detection in the context of transient ischemic attacks cannot be emphasized. Although the symptoms of a TIA may subside on their own, they are a warning sign for underlying vascular problems that require prompt attention.

Early detection allows medical professionals to evaluate the patient's risk factors, start preventive measures, and create a customized treatment plan to reduce the risk of a more severe stroke later on. Additionally, it empowers patients to modify their lifestyle and follow prescribed guidelines, promoting a proactive approach to vascular health.

A thorough comprehension of the Transient Ischemic Attack includes its definition, causes, symptoms, and the critical importance of early detection. By dissecting the complexities surrounding TIA, individuals, and healthcare professionals can work together to minimize the effects of this brief but significant neurological event.

CHAPTER TWO

THE TIA MEDICAL ENVIRONMENT

MEDICAL TESTING AND DIAGNOSIS

Transient Ischemic Attacks (TIAs) are diagnosed by a thorough review of the patient's medical history, symptoms, and physical examination. Diagnostic tests are frequently used by medical professionals to verify the existence of a TIA and determine potential risk factors. Imaging studies, like computed tomography (CT) scans and magnetic resonance imaging (MRIs), are essential for visualizing the brain and identifying abnormalities or signs of ischemia.

Vascular imaging, like carotid ultrasound or angiography, may be utilized to evaluate blood flow and identify possible sources of emboli or stenosis.

DISTINGUISHING A TIA FROM A STROKE

Differentiating between a transient ischemic attack (TIA) and a full-blown stroke is critical for the proper medical management of both conditions. Although both are characterized by a temporary disruption of blood flow to the brain, TIAs are characterized by transient symptoms that usually go away in less than 24 hours. Moreover, TIAs do not involve persistent neurological deficits, unlike strokes, where symptoms frequently persist.

Advanced imaging techniques and comprehensive clinical assessments help healthcare professionals make this critical distinction, which in turn helps them develop targeted treatment plans and preventive measures.

CONSULTATION WITH MEDICAL SPECIALISTS

Considering the severity of TIAs and their correlation with a higher risk of subsequent strokes, patients must seek professional consultation as soon as possible. Physicians, neurologists, and vascular specialists can work together to evaluate the patient's general health, identify risk factors, and customize interventions. An essential part of consultations is patient education, which helps patients comprehend the importance of

TIAs, take prescribed medications, and modify their lifestyles in ways that support long-term vascular health.

INTERVENTIONS AND TREATMENT OPTIONS:

Treatment for transient ischemic attacks (TIAs) is a multimodal strategy that tries to prevent recurrence and minimize the risk of stroke. Physicians can prescribe antiplatelet drugs, like aspirin or clopidogrel, to prevent blood clots from forming and lower the risk of ischemic episodes.

Modifiable risk factors, like diabetes, hypertension, and hyperlipidemia, must also be addressed with medication and lifestyle changes. Surgical procedures, like carotid endarterectomy or angioplasty with stenting, are sometimes advised to relieve vascular blockages and improve blood flow.

Comprehending the medical environment surrounding transient ischemic attacks requires an all-encompassing strategy that includes diagnosis, distinguishing them from strokes, consulting with medical professionals, and offering a variety of treatment options and interventions. By fusing cutting-edge diagnostic tools with cooperative healthcare initiatives, TIAs can be effectively managed, the risk of recurrent strokes can be decreased, and overall patient outcomes can be enhanced.

CHAPTER THREE

CHANGES IN LIFESTYLE TO PREVENT TIAS

HEALTHY DIET

It is impossible to overestimate the significance of lifestyle modifications in the prevention of Transient Ischemic Attacks (TIAs). These changes are essential in lowering the risk factors linked to TIAs and improving general cardiovascular health. People who adopt a healthier lifestyle can improve their overall well-being and significantly reduce their chance of suffering a TIA.

A heart-healthy diet full of fruits, vegetables, whole grains, and lean proteins helps control blood pressure and cholesterol levels.

Reducing saturated and trans fats is important to minimize the buildup of plaque in arteries, which lowers the risk of blood clots that may lead to TIAs. Dietary guidelines are essential for preventing TIAs because nutrition plays a critical role in maintaining vascular health.

EXERCISE AND PHYSICAL ACTIVITY

Exercise and physical activity are essential parts of a strategy to prevent TIAs. Being physically active regularly helps maintain a healthy weight, improves cardiovascular health, and controls blood pressure. Aerobic exercises, like swimming, jogging, or walking, improve blood circulation and lower the risk of blood clots, which in turn lowers the risk of TIAs.

The impact of stress, which is known to increase the risk of TIAs, must be mitigated. Prolonged stress can raise blood pressure and have a detrimental effect on vascular health overall. Mindfulness, meditation, and yoga are some of the practices that can effectively lower stress levels and improve emotional well-being, which in turn increases the body's resistance to TIAs.

ALCOHOL MODERATION

Alcohol moderation is also advised, as excessive alcohol consumption can contribute to elevated blood pressure and increase the risk of TIAs. Moderated alcohol intake is a prudent step in maintaining vascular health and reducing TIA risk. Quitting smoking is a crucial lifestyle change for preventing TIAs, as it damages blood vessels and increases the risk of blood clot formation. Individuals who quit smoking significantly decrease their chances of experiencing TIAs and improve their overall cardiovascular health.

Lifestyle changes are crucial to preventing TIAs. People can actively lower the risk factors linked to TIAs and support long-term cardiovascular well-being by following dietary recommendations, exercising frequently, managing stress, giving up smoking, and consuming alcohol in moderation. These lifestyle changes also create the groundwork for a happier, healthier, and longer life.

CHAPTER FOUR

MEDICATION ADMINISTRATION
AN OVERVIEW OF TRANSIENT ISCHEMIC ATTACK (TIA) MEDICATION

Transient Ischemic Attack (TIA) is a condition that is characterized by a temporary disruption of blood flow to the brain. The main objective of medication therapy for TIA is to reduce the risk factors associated with vascular events and prevent future strokes.

Various classes of medications are commonly prescribed to address different aspects of TIA management. These include blood pressure management agents, cholesterol-lowering medications, and antiplatelet and anticoagulant medications.

ANTICOAGULANT AND ANTIPLATELET DRUGS

Cornerstone therapies in the prevention of recurrent transient ischemic attacks (TIAs) and strokes include antiplatelet and anticoagulant medications. Since the pathophysiology of TIAs involves platelet aggregation and blood clot formation, antiplatelet drugs like aspirin are commonly prescribed; aspirin inhibits platelet aggregation and lowers the risk of clot formation, preventing the occlusion of blood vessels in the brain. In some cases, anticoagulant medications, such as warfarin or direct oral anticoagulants (DOACs), may be taken into consideration to further reduce the risk of blood clots.

CONTROLLING BLOOD PRESSURE

Tight blood pressure control not only addresses the immediate risk associated with TIA but also contributes to long-term vascular health. Antihypertensive medications are frequently prescribed to control blood pressure levels because hypertension is a significant risk factor for cerebrovascular events.

Medications like angiotensin-converting enzyme (ACE) inhibitors, angiotensin II receptor blockers (ARBs), beta-blockers, and diuretics are commonly used to achieve and maintain optimal blood pressure.

DRUGS THAT LOWER CHOLESTEROL

High levels of low-density lipoprotein (LDL) cholesterol are known risk factors for stroke and transient ischemic attacks (TIAs).

Statins, which lower cholesterol, are essential for controlling lipid profiles and lowering the amount of atherosclerotic plaque in blood vessels because they prevent the synthesis of new cholesterol, which lowers LDL levels and helps to stabilize atherosclerotic plaques. By treating hyperlipidemia, these drugs also help to lower the overall risk for vascular events, including TIAs.

Drug therapy for transient ischemic attacks (TIAs) is complex and targets various facets of the underlying pathology.

Blood pressure control agents regulate hypertension, antiplatelet and anticoagulant medications prevent clot formation, and cholesterol-lowering medications treat dyslipidemia.

When combined, these pharmacological interventions attempt to offer a comprehensive approach to TIA prevention, ultimately lowering the risk of recurrent transient ischemic events and promoting long-term vascular health.

CHAPTER FIVE

OVERCOMING PSYCHOLOGICAL AND EMOTIONAL OBSTACLES

HANDLING THE EMOTIONAL EFFECT

Life is a complex tapestry of events, and people will inevitably run into emotional obstacles that can be both terrifying and transforming. Handling the emotional fallout calls for a sophisticated strategy that recognizes the range of feelings and the individuality of each person's reaction. Cultivating emotional resilience—the capacity to overcome hardship and preserve mental health—is one essential component.

Mindfulness is a useful coping technique that entails being fully present in the moment without passing judgment. Through non-reactively observing their feelings, mindfulness practices—like meditation and deep breathing exercises—allow people to have a better knowledge of their inner moods. Furthermore, pursuing joyful and fulfilling pursuits can function as a potent antidote to mental suffering by providing a break from difficulties and encouraging an optimistic outlook.

Additionally, getting expert assistance through counseling or therapy can give you useful coping mechanisms for handling emotional upheaval. Professional therapists provide support in managing difficult feelings, encouraging self-awareness, and creating coping strategies. Acknowledging one's vulnerability and embracing help is an essential step on the path to emotional well-being.

NETWORKS AND SUPPORT SYSTEMS

To overcome emotional and psychological obstacles, human connection is essential. Building and maintaining networks and support systems is crucial to establishing a safety net in trying circumstances. A strong foundation for emotional support can be formed by the empathy, comprehension, and helpful advice that family, friends, and coworkers can provide.

Establishing robust support networks requires open communication. Speaking with someone one can trust about one's feelings and worries helps one feel less alone and less burdened by emotional difficulties. Furthermore, empathetic support networks and active listening foster a helpful environment in which people feel validated and heard.

Online forums and social media platforms are also important sources of support in the digital era. Through virtual platforms, people can connect with others who share their interests and are going through similar issues. This helps people feel less alone, which is typically associated with emotional struggles and can provide a sense of belonging. Creating a broad network of support guarantees that people have different people to turn to when they need help.

CONSIDERING MENTAL HEALTH

The emotional, psychological, and social facets of well-being are all included in the complex concept of mental health. Understanding how these factors interact and approaching mental health issues holistically is essential. Recognizing that mental health is a spectrum on which individuals may fall at various places destigmatizes asking for assistance and encourages taking an active role in one's well-being.

Maintaining mental health requires regular self-evaluation and self-care. To avoid burnout, this entails identifying early indicators of suffering, giving self-care activities a top priority, and setting up appropriate boundaries. Integrating stress-reduction strategies, such as physical activity, getting enough sleep, and practicing calm, can improve mental health in general.

The de-stigmatization of mental health discussions is essential to building a culture that is accepting and helpful. Promoting open communication about mental health issues reduces stigma and increases empathy and understanding, which in turn helps people seek the care they need. In schools, businesses, and communities, highlighting the significance of mental health education helps to foster a culture that values and gives psychological well-being priority.

CHAPTER SIX

TAKING CHARGE OF YOUR EDUCATION

FINDING OUT MORE ABOUT YOUR HEALTH

Developing knowledge and understanding in a variety of areas of your life, especially about health and wellbeing, is a transforming process that goes hand in hand with empowering yourself via education. An essential first step in this approach is to educate yourself on your disease.

You may demystify the intricacies surrounding your health condition and improve your ability to make educated decisions about your care by being knowledgeable about its particular. Knowing the nature, symptoms, and accessible therapies of any medical condition—be it chronic sickness, mental health issue, or otherwise—can greatly empower you to take an active role in managing your health.

STAYING CURRENT WITH DEVELOPMENTS AND RESEARCH

Keeping up with research and breakthroughs is essential for learning about the latest developments in medical science, in addition to comprehending your situation. Healthcare is a dynamic field where novel treatments, therapies, and breakthroughs are always being produced by continuing study. Keeping your knowledge base up to date enables you to investigate new avenues that could expand your options for treatment. By empowering you to ask relevant questions, participate actively in treatment plan conversations, and interact more effectively with healthcare providers, this proactive approach not only keeps you informed but also gives you a sense of empowerment.

One of the most important components of education-based self-empowerment is speaking up for your health. This entails taking an active role in your healthcare journey, standing up for your rights, and making sure that you are heard when decisions are being made.

Getting involved with healthcare practitioners, communicating your preferences and concerns, and enquiring about treatment alternatives are all part of being an advocate for your health. It also entails keeping up with healthcare policies and activities so that you may support more general issues that could affect both your well-being and the well-being of those who are going through comparable difficulties.

SPEAKING UP FOR YOUR HEALTH

Education may empower people in more ways than just academics; it can also be used in real-world situations and to involve them in the healthcare system. You actively create your road to well-being by being knowledgeable about your illness, staying up to date on research and speaking up for your health. Taking the initiative can help you live a more satisfying and powerful life in which you are in charge of decisions about your health and actively participate in the continuing conversation about improvements and practices in healthcare.

CHAPTER SEVEN

CONSTRUCTING AN ALL-INCLUSIVE CARE PLAN

WORKING TOGETHER WITH YOUR MEDICAL TEAM

Working together with your healthcare team is essential to creating a complete treatment plan. To meet your specific needs, this team usually consists of doctors, nurses, specialists, and other medical experts. Successful collaborations are built on effective communication, which makes sure that everyone is aware of each other's goals, treatment preferences, and state of health. You can actively engage in decision-making processes by having open discussions and offering insightful feedback that will help define your care plan.

In addition, the teamwork involves not just medical professionals but also those in your close circle of support, including friends, family, and caregivers. Their participation is essential for offering psychological support, arranging for useful help, and improving general well-being. A comprehensive strategy that takes into accounts not only the physical elements of your health but also its social and emotional components is produced by the collaboration of healthcare experts with your personal support network.

DEVELOPING A CUSTOMIZED CARE PLAN

A customized care plan is made to accommodate your unique health requirements, preferences, and situation. It recognizes the individuality of your medical history, lifestyle, and personal objectives, going beyond a one-size-fits-all strategy. A complete evaluation of your health situation, which includes a review of your medical history, results of any diagnostic tests, and a consideration of any underlying causes or chronic diseases, is the first step in creating such a strategy.

When your healthcare team collaborates to create solutions that reflect your beliefs and preferences, collaboration comes into play. This could entail a mix of therapeutic interventions, lifestyle changes, and pharmaceutical management.

Your active participation in the decision-making process transforms the care plan into a joint effort that encourages a sense of commitment to the suggested tactics and ownership.

An individualized treatment plan also considers the ever-changing character of health. It needs to be adaptive and flexible enough to alter your health. Frequent reviews and modifications are crucial elements that guarantee the strategy stays applicable and efficient in meeting your changing needs over time.

FREQUENT OBSERVATION AND FOLLOW-UP

A comprehensive care plan must include monitoring and follow-up since they act as regular checkpoints to assess the plan's efficacy and make any required modifications. Vital signs, test findings, and symptomatology are examples of important health indicators that are tracked regularly to evaluate progress and quickly spot possible problems.

Your healthcare team's follow-up appointments offer a chance for cooperative conversations when you can voice any concerns, ask questions, and share comments. These meetings serve as a forum for adjusting the care plan in light of your changing requirements and preferences, as well as a way to assess the success of interventions.

A proactive approach to managing your health is fostered by regular contact between you and your healthcare staff. It makes it possible to identify any issues early, makes preventive actions easier, and strengthens the bond between you and your medical professionals. The care plan becomes a dynamic and adaptable instrument that maximizes its effectiveness in improving your overall well-being via consistent monitoring and follow-up.

CHAPTER EIGHT

OVERCOMING OBSTACLES AND FAILURES

DEALING WITH SETBACKS AND PROBLEMS

Life is an erratic path full of turns and turns, and it frequently throws us into difficult and depressing setbacks and problems. The capacity to confront and overcome challenges is essential for personal development and well-being, regardless of whether they are brought on by a personal setback, a professional setback, or an unforeseen life event. Overcoming setbacks requires adopting an attitude that is more concerned with growth and learning than with concentrating on the drawbacks.

When faced with obstacles, it's critical to conduct an unbiased analysis of the problem, pinpointing the underlying causes and comprehending the elements that contributed to the difficulty. This process of self-examination can yield insightful information that forms the basis for creating practical solutions to the problems at hand. People can develop a proactive, upbeat mindset that empowers them to go on with resilience by accepting setbacks as chances for learning and progression.

ADAPTIVE STRATEGIES FOR DAILY LIVING

These are crucial tools that enable people to deal with life's challenges in a flexible and inventive manner. Because life is dynamic, unforeseen changes will inevitably occur. Creating an attitude that welcomes change and uncertainty is essential to developing adaptive tactics because it enables prompt adjustments in response to changing conditions. The capacity to create and carry out adaptive strategies is essential whether adjusting to a new work environment, managing relationships, or dealing with health issues.

To effectively adapt, people should cultivate a growth mindset, which sees obstacles as chances for growth and learning. Adopting a growth mindset promotes ongoing education and the development of new abilities, encouraging a proactive attitude to conquering obstacles in daily life. Furthermore, being conscious and in the present moment might help people become more adaptable by allowing them to react to changing circumstances deliberately rather than impulsively.

ADAPTABILITY AND MENTAL HARDINESS

A person's capacity to overcome adversity and face obstacles head-on with fortitude and resolve depends heavily on their resilience and mental toughness. The ability to bounce back from hardship, adjust to change, and keep a good attitude in the face of adversity are all components of resilience. It is a trait that can be developed by going through challenging situations that present chances for personal development.

Resilience and mental toughness go hand in hand; mental toughness is the capacity to endure hardship. Developing a robust mindset, attention, and a strong sense of self-discipline are all necessary for developing mental toughness. With high mental toughness, people can remain composed under duress; remain inspired in the face of failures, and keep going for their objectives despite difficulties.

Resilience and mental toughness must be developed via deliberate work and a dedication to personal development. The development of these vital traits can be facilitated by taking part in activities that push and challenge one's talents, looking for assistance from a strong social network, and keeping an optimistic attitude on life. Ultimately, people can overcome obstacles and come out stronger on the other side by accepting setbacks as opportunities for growth, using adaptive methods, and building resilience and mental toughness.